Endomorph Fat Loss Program

A Complete Nutrition and Workout Plan for Endomorphs to Burn
Fat and Build Lean Muscle

B. TERZA

© [2024] B. TERZA. All rights reserved.

No part of this publication may be reproduced, distributed, or transmitted in any form or by any means, including photocopying, recording, or other electronic or mechanical methods, without the prior written permission of the author, except in the case of brief quotations embodied in reviews and certain noncommercial uses permitted by copyright law.

Endomorph Fat Loss Program

Contents

INTRODUCTION 5

Welcome to Endomorph Fat Loss! 5

Endomorph Physiology Science 6

(Section 1:) 9

Understanding the Endomorph Body Type..9

1. What Characterizes an Endomorph? 9

2. Difficulties of Endomorphism...11

3. Making Use of the Endomorph Advantage 13

CALL TO ACTION 16

(Section 2:) 17

Formulating the Ideal Endomorph Diet. 17

4. Plan for the endomorph diet...17

5 Complex carbs, lean proteins, and healthy fats. 19

6. Templates for weekly meal planning 22

7. sporadic fasting 23

How Intermittent Fasting Can Aid in Fat Loss 24

Best Times and Methods for Fasting...24

(SECTION 3:) 26

Exercises Particular to Endomorphs..26

8. Resistance Training's Significance 26

9. Exercise Splits to Gain Muscle and Lose Fat..28

10. Examples of Exercises...30

11. Getting Moving Outside of the Gym 32

How to Stay Active During Days of Rest..32

(SECTION 4:) 34

Endomorph Training Cheats and Techniques 34

12. The Mind-Muscle Connection: The Secret to Successful Exercise......34

13. Lifting Techniques for Better Results 35

Tricks to Make the Most of Every Workout 36

14. Cardiology for Endomorphs 37

Endomorph Fat Loss Program

(SECTION 5:) 40

Maintaining Direction and Preventing Stagnation 40

15. Overcoming Typical Roadblocks 40

Tips for Staying Motivated on a Mental and Emotional Level 41

16. Monitoring Your Development 42

How to Modify Your Initiative for Ongoing Outcomes 43

(Section 6:) 45

A Long-Term Strategy for Fat Loss 45

17. Preserving Your Outcomes 45

How to Add Carbs Back in Without Putting on Weight 46

18. Endomorphs and Health Throughout Life 48

Managing a Healthy Metabolism Over Time 49

In summary: 51

Consider Your Journey Again 51

Creating New Routines 52

Creating Future Objectives 53

Building a Community of Support 54

Sustaining Prolonged Achievement 54

Last Words 55

CALL TO ACTION 56

INTRODUCTION

Welcome to Endomorph Fat Loss!

Thank you for beginning your quest to enhance your fitness and overall health! Welcome to the Endomorph Fat Loss Program, the beginning of your particular journey. You are not the only one who has struggled to grow lean muscle and lose fat. Many persons who identify as endomorphic face obstacles that sometimes appear insurmountable. However, this program is designed specifically for you, leveraging the power of tailored nutrition programs and effective exercise routines to help you achieve your fitness goals.

This essay is intended to help you understand your body and what it requires to thrive, not just lose weight. Here, we'll go deeply into the specifics of your body type, find the best practices for you, and provide you with the tools you need to take control of your fitness journey.

Understanding Your Body: What Does Being an Endomorph Mean?
Before we go into the program's subtleties, let's first define what it means to be an endomorph. Ectomorph, mesomorph, and endomorph are the three most popular body type categories used in fitness and nutrition. Each type has unique characteristics, advantages, and downsides.

Endomorph Fat Loss Program

Endomorphs typically have softer, rounder bodies with a larger percentage of body fat. You may notice that your shoulders are narrow, your hips are broader, and your lower body carries the majority of your weight. Furthermore, if you have a slower metabolism than others, weight loss may be more difficult for you. Nonetheless, recognizing these traits is the first step toward harnessing your unique physiology for optimal fat loss.

The good news is that, despite their genetic proclivity to store fat, endomorphs have incredible strength training and muscle building potential. Endomorphs are fantastic weightlifters and resistance trainers, so with the right technique, you may transform your body into a stronger, thinner version of yourself.

Endomorph Physiology Science

Understanding the science behind your body's physiology will help you achieve your fat loss goals. Endomorphs frequently experience hormonal fluctuations, which impact how their bodies absorb food. According to research, those with a higher proportion of body fat may have altered insulin sensitivity and hormonal profiles, which could affect fat accumulation and energy usage.

Insulin, a key hormone in metabolism, regulates blood sugar levels and fat storage. Insulin sensitivity may be reduced in many endomorphs, causing difficulty managing blood sugar and increasing fat storage. This is a transitory condition, and you may improve your body's ability to use insulin by adopting the necessary dietary and lifestyle changes.

Endomorph Fat Loss Program

Metabolic mechanisms also affect endomorphic physiology. Endomorphs often have a slower metabolic rate than other body types, meaning they burn calories more slowly. This is why endomorphs frequently discover that a one-size-fits-all approach to exercise and dieting fails. To burn fat and increase lean muscle mass, your body need a personalized strategy that takes into consideration these metabolic oddities.

Furthermore, your genetic composition has a significant impact on how your body responds to various diets and exercise programs. Learning about these inherited variables will allow you to adjust your training routine more precisely. Understanding your individual physiological composition allows you to focus on the strategies that will work best for you.

Setting realistic expectations for muscle gain, fat loss, and body composition Setting realistic goals for yourself is critical as you begin this journey. Fat loss is a nonlinear process with ups and downs. Many people quit up when they don't see immediate results, but it's vital to remember that growing muscle and decreasing fat requires time and commitment.

Determine your own definition of success first. Rather than focusing just on the number on the scale, consider other indicators of success such as increased strength, vitality, and overall well-being. Keeping track of your small victories can inspire and motivate you as you progress.

This method seeks to create a sustainable lifestyle that promotes fat loss and lean muscle gain. This includes promoting healthy nutrition, effective activity, and a positive perspective. Accept the process and remember that small changes might build up over time.

Finally, don't be hesitant to seek assistance and advice while traveling. Being in the company of positive people, whether through friends, a personal trainer, or a fitness club, can make a significant difference.

(Section 1:)

Understanding the Endomorph Body Type

1. What Characterizes an Endomorph?

When addressing body types, we usually refer to psychologist William Sheldon's somatotype classification system, which he developed in the 1940s. This classification identifies three main body types: ectomorph, mesomorph, and endomorph. This section will look at what defines an endomorph, emphasizing its distinguishing characteristics and how it differs from other body types.

Features include body composition, fat storage, and metabolism.

Endomorphs typically have a soft, round body shape with a larger hip and waist circumference and a naturally higher body fat percentage. If you struggle to lose weight or if your body tends to acquire weight quickly, you may be an endomorph.

Endomorphs have the following distinguishing characteristics:

Endomorphs typically have a larger rib cage, wider hips, and a broader frame. This body type lacks the definite muscle tone observed in other body types,

Endomorph Fat Loss Program

causing it to appear softer and rounder. Body fat is often distributed in the thighs, hips, and stomach areas.

Metabolism is one of an endomorph's most distinguishing features. Endomorphs have slower metabolic rates than ectomorphs and mesomorphs, hence they burn calories less efficiently. This sluggish metabolism can make it difficult to lose weight and lead to an increased tendency to store fat.

Endomorphs are genetically predisposed to accumulating fat, which can have both favorable and negative consequences. They can grow muscle faster than other body types, but they have a harder time reducing fat. Endomorphs must employ specific nutritional strategies to combat the body's tendency to store calories as fat.

Ectomorphs and Mesomorphs, two more body types, differ from endomorphs.

Understanding the differences between endomorphs and mesomorphs might shed light on the unique challenges and advantages connected with this body type:

Ectomorphs are distinguished by a thin, slender build with small hips and shoulders. Their metabolism is fast, allowing them to burn calories quickly. Ectomorphs' high metabolic rate makes it harder for them to gain muscle mass, however it can help with fat loss.

Mesomorphs are more athletic and muscular, having broad shoulders and a narrow waist. They gain muscle and lose fat more easily than endomorphs. They

Endomorph Fat Loss Program

respond effectively to both strength and aerobic training due to their balanced metabolism.

In contrast, endomorphs have a unique set of characteristics. While they may struggle with fat loss, their body composition frequently promotes muscle growth, making them ideal candidates for strength training. Understanding these variations is critical for designing exercise and food routines that are most beneficial for your body type.

2. Difficulties of Endomorphism

Every body type faces unique challenges, but endomorphs usually struggle with muscle gain and fat loss. Understanding these barriers is critical to successfully overcoming them.

Why It Can Be Difficult to Lose Fat

Endomorphs may find it particularly challenging to reduce weight due to their unique metabolic profile. Here are some explanations for this.

Endomorphs often have a slower metabolic rate, as previously mentioned. This suggests that they may not lose as much fat as ectomorphs or mesomorphs, even if they consume fewer calories. When you put up your best efforts and the scale remains stationary, it might be frustrating.

Insulin Resistance: Insulin resistance is a condition that many endomorphs experience, in which their bodies become less responsive to insulin. This may

Endomorph Fat Loss Program

result in increased levels of circulating insulin, which promotes fat storage. As a result, even a low carbohydrate consumption can impede weight loss efforts.

Endomorphs have an inherited predisposition to fat storage, particularly around the waist. Because even minor dietary changes might induce weight gain, this can create a vicious cycle of frustration.

Motivational obstacles and psychological barriers.

Being an endomorph may present psychological challenges on par with physical issues. Here are a few common mental obstacles:

Poor Body Image: Losing weight can lead to feelings of inadequacy and a negative body image. Endomorphs may be frustrated with the size and shape of their bodies, which can sap their confidence and motivation to exercise.

Comparison with Others: It's easy to fall into the trap of comparing oneself to others, especially those who seem to lose weight effortlessly. This may exacerbate psychological problems by instilling feelings of jealously and discouragement.

Fear of Failure: It can be difficult to commit to a new program if one is afraid of failing owing to previous dieting experiences. Endomorphs may be hesitant to start a new workout plan due to previous setbacks.

It is critical to cultivate an optimistic attitude in order to overcome these psychological difficulties. Rather than focusing solely on the scale, consider your accomplishments and talents. Celebrate your non-scale accomplishments, like as increased vigor, physical prowess, and overall wellbeing.

3. Making Use of the Endomorph Advantage

Despite the challenges that endomorphs face, there are certain advantages that can be used to achieve optimal fat loss and muscle building. You can turn the situation to your favor by focusing on your unique skills.

Endomorphs excel at building muscle and strength.

Being able to grow muscle and engage in strength training is one of the primary advantages of being an endomorph. Here's how to make use of this benefit:

Endomorphs have a larger ratio of muscular mass to body fat than other body types, which allows them to gain strength more quickly. Their ability to successfully convert dietary protein into muscle tissue is the explanation behind this.

Progressive Overload: Incorporating progressive overload into strength training can produce astonishing results. This involves progressively increasing the amount of weight you can lift. Lifting heavier weights encourages muscle growth and increases your resting metabolic rate, allowing you to burn more calories while at rest.

Compound motions: Endomorphs are usually competent at complex motions that require several muscle groups. Squats, deadlifts, bench presses, and rows are all effective muscle-building workouts. To get the most out of your training, make these workouts a primary priority.

Metabolic Changes to Remove Sticky Fat

Endomorphs can make the following distinct metabolic changes to help combat the problems of fat loss:

High-Intensity Interval Training (HIIT): Incorporating HIIT into your training routine will help you lose weight faster. HIIT is made up of short bursts of intense activity followed by rest intervals. It has been shown that this type of exercise improves insulin sensitivity and metabolism, allowing endomorphs to reduce stubborn fat.

Strategic Carb Cycling: Because endomorphs have a tendency to build fat, carb cycling can be an effective strategy. Rotating between high-carb and low-carb days allows you to fuel your workouts while also encouraging fat reduction. Increase your carbohydrate intake to help you stay energized on training days. Reduce carbohydrates on rest days to improve fat burning.

Keeping an Eye on Macronutrient Intake: Endomorphs often benefit from eating more protein because it preserves muscle mass and promotes fat loss. The macronutrient ratio should be around 40% protein, 30% fat, and 30% carbohydrates. This balance can enhance muscle growth and improve metabolic processes.

In summary:

Endomorph Fat Loss Program

Understanding the endomorph body type is critical to developing a program that effectively decreases body fat while increasing muscle mass. If you are aware of your unique qualities, advantages, and challenges, you may tailor your fitness journey to meet your own needs. Accept the benefits of your body type and remember that a combination of mental toughness, dietary strategies, and physical exercise may be required for success. You may achieve your fitness goals and transform your body in a sustainable way if you are devoted to the process and take the right approach.

CALL TO ACTION

Thank you for reading!

I'd like to personally thank you for taking the time to read my work. I really appreciate your time and effort, and I hope this book has provided you with valuable success tools and insights.

Your feedback is really useful to me as I grow as a writer. I would love to hear your feedback, whether positive or negative, so that I may develop and make future works even more useful and fascinating.

I humbly request that you offer an honest review if you found this book worthwhile or if you believe anything may be improved. Your counsel will help me not only improve, but also become a better person.

Thank you again for your support, and I look forward to hearing from you!

SINCERLY

(Section 2:)

Formulating the Ideal Endomorph Diet.

4. Plan for the endomorph diet.

Understanding an endomorph's unique physiology and metabolic needs is critical to creating the ideal diet plan for them. The goal is to design a nutrition plan that promotes fat loss while retaining lean muscle mass. This section discusses the macronutrient breakdown, meal frequency, and timing, all of which are crucial for optimal results.

Macronutrient breakdown: High fat, moderate protein, low to moderate carbohydrates.

Endomorphs require a tailored macronutrient breakdown to properly shed fat while maintaining muscle mass. Here's how you should organize your diet:

Endomorphs require a high protein diet since it helps them retain muscle build while also promoting fat loss. Try to acquire 30-40% of your total calories from protein. Plant-based meals like beans and tofu, as well as lean meats like fish, fowl, and turkey, should be your primary sources of nutrition.

Endomorph Fat Loss Program

Moderate Fat: Healthy fats are essential for hormonal synthesis and overall wellness. Try to acquire 25-30% of your daily calories from fat-rich foods such as avocados, nuts, seeds, and olive oil. Incorporating these fats into your diet improves hormone balance and satiety, which is particularly advantageous for endomorphs.

Low to Moderate carbs: Endomorphs frequently have a reduced carb tolerance, which, if consumed in excess, can lead to fat storage. As a result, aim to take 30-40% of your total calories from complex carbohydrates. Limit processed sweets and simple carbohydrates and focus on nutrient-dense foods like whole grains, vegetables, and legumes.

This macronutrient split supports the specific demands of endomorphs, encouraging fat loss while delivering the energy required for exercises and daily activities.

The timing and frequency of meals have a significant effect on fat loss and metabolic rate. Endomorph techniques include the following:

Regular Meal Schedule: Eating on a regular schedule will help you control your blood sugar levels and avoid overeating when you are hungry. Aim for four to six small meals per day, with a mix of complex carbohydrates, healthy fats, and protein at each.

Pre- and post-workout nutrition: To achieve the best outcomes and recovery, fuel your body both before and after exercise. Try eating a high-protein meal or snack 30-60 minutes before working out. Prioritize protein and a few excellent

Endomorph Fat Loss Program

carbohydrates to help with muscle repair and glycogen replenishment after a workout.

Mindful Eating: By paying attention to hunger cues, you can improve digestion and reduce overeating. Endomorphs benefit the most from eating more slowly, enjoying their meal, and paying heed to their bodies' fullness cues.

Making the right meal selections is critical for achieving maximum fat loss and lean muscle gain. This section provides useful grocery lists and highlights the best foods for endomorphs.

5 Complex carbs, lean proteins, and healthy fats.

To achieve your fitness goals, you must eat the right meals. The following is a summary of the best foods for endomorphs:

Lean Proteins: Focus on high-quality, low-fat protein sources. Good choices include:

Breast of chicken.
Turkey
Fish (including tuna and salmon)
Whites and Eggs
Greek yogurt
Legumes (lentils, beans)
Complex Carbohydrates: These are essential for exercise and provide long-term energy. Choose to:

Endomorph Fat Loss Program

Quinoa
Grains of brown rice
yams
Whole wheat pasta and bread.
oats
vegetables and leafy greens.
excellent Fats: To support hormone balance and satiety, include the following excellent fat sources in your diet.

Avocados
Nuts and seeds, such as flaxseed, chia seeds, and almonds
Olive oil
fatty fish, such mackerel and sardines.
Sample Grocery Lists to Build Lean Muscle and Burn Fat

Making a grocery list might help you streamline your shopping trip and focus on healthier options. This is a sample grocery list created with endomorphs in mind.

Proteins:

Breast of chicken.
Salmon
Eggs
Greek yogurt
lentils

Endomorph Fat Loss Program

Glucose:

Quinoa
Grains of brown rice
yams
Sprouts
broccoli
Lipids:

Avocado
Almonds
Chia seeds
Olive oil
Munchies:

Hummus (to dip vegetables into)
Protein bars (select those with less sugar)
Berries with Greek yogurt
A well-rounded grocery list can help you achieve your dietary goals while also encouraging healthy eating, making it easier to stick to your endomorph diet plan.

Recipes

Meal planning is an effective strategy for muscle gain and weight loss. This section provides simple recipes and templates to help endomorphs eat healthily while enjoying it.

Endomorph Fat Loss Program

6. Templates for weekly meal planning

Making a weekly meal plan will help you stay focused and organized. Here's a basic template to get you started:

Weekly Meal Plan Example:

Lunch: Monday through Thursday, Friday, Saturday, and Sunday
Breakfast options include avocado toast with eggs, omelette with vegetables, overnight oats with berries, Greek yogurt with almonds, and protein smoothie.

Fruit and nut butter snack; carrot sticks and hummus; protein bar; cottage cheese and fruit; celery with peanut butter; mixed nuts; dark chocolate and berries

Lunch options include stir-fried chicken, grilled vegetable wrap, lentil soup, turkey wrap, and Quinoa and black bean bowl.

Snack: whole-grain crackers with cheese and guacamole; rice cakes with nut butter; hard-boiled eggs; and Greek yogurt.

Dinner options include shrimp tacos, turkey meatballs, zucchini noodles with marinara, baked chicken and broccoli, and grilled steak and asparagus.
Simple and Quick Recipes for Active Endomorphs

To make meal preparation easier and ensure that your meals are pleasurable, try these simple recipes:

Endomorph Fat Loss Program

Rich in Protein Omelette

Ingredients: feta cheese, bell peppers, spinach, and two eggs.
Directions: Beat eggs and transfer to a heated skillet. Add the bell peppers and spinach. Cook until set, sprinkle feta cheese, fold, and serve.
Quinoa Bowl

Ingredients: Cooked quinoa, cherry tomatoes, cucumber, feta cheese, and olive oil.
Directions: In a bowl, combine all ingredients and toss with olive oil. Season with pepper and salt.
Grilled Chicken Wrap

Ingredients: avocado, lettuce, grilled chicken breast, and whole grain wrap.
Directions: Arrange all components in the wrap, firmly roll, and have a wholesome lunch that can be had on the go.
wholesome smoothie

Ingredients: 1 cup almond milk, 1 banana, 1 cup spinach, and 1 scoop protein powder.
Instructions: For a cool post-workout snack, blend all ingredients until smooth.

7. sporadic fasting

Recent years have seen a rise in the popularity of intermittent fasting (IF), which is especially advantageous for endomorphs. This section looks at the

Endomorph Fat Loss Program

optimal fasting windows and methods to think about, as well as how IF can help with fat loss.

How Intermittent Fasting Can Aid in Fat Loss

Cycling between eating and fasting phases is known as intermittent fasting. For endomorphs, this strategy may be helpful for a number of reasons:

Increased Fat Oxidation: Fasting intervals have been shown to enhance fat oxidation, which encourages fat loss while maintaining muscle mass. The body uses fat that has been stored as fuel during fasting, which can lower body fat percentage.

Increased Insulin Sensitivity: By increasing insulin sensitivity, intermittent fasting can facilitate the body's efficient use of glucose. This is especially crucial for endomorphs because they are more likely to experience insulin resistance.

Simplified Meal Planning: Meal planning can be made easier by restricting the eating window. This can help endomorphs focus on nutrient-dense foods and lessen the urge for harmful snacks.

Best Times and Methods for Fasting

Here are some well-liked techniques to look at if you're thinking about introducing intermittent fasting into your daily routine:

Endomorph Fat Loss Program

16/8 Method: This protocol calls for an 8-hour window during which food is consumed after 16 hours of fasting. You may, for instance, eat between 12 and 8 p.m. This strategy is adaptable and works well with a variety of lifestyles.

(SECTION 3:)

Exercises Particular to Endomorphs

8. Resistance Training's Significance

Why Endomorphs Need to Lift Weights to Lose Fat

Resistance training is essential for endomorphs to lose fat and improve their overall body composition. Given this body type's slower metabolism and increased propensity to accumulate fat, weightlifting is a crucial part of any successful fitness regimen. This is the reason why:

Muscle Mass and Metabolism: Resistance training raises your resting metabolic rate (RMR) by helping you gain lean muscle mass. This implies that your body continues to burn calories while at rest, which aids in overall fat loss. A more desirable body composition can be achieved by increasing muscular mass, as endomorphs frequently suffer with excess body fat.

Hormonal Balance: Resistance exercise affects the synthesis of growth hormone and testosterone, two hormones essential for fat loss. These hormones are essential for endomorphs trying to lose excess weight because they encourage fat burning and muscle building.

Endomorph Fat Loss Program

Increased Insulin Sensitivity: Lifting weights on a regular basis increases insulin sensitivity, which lowers the chance of fat storage and improves your body's ability to use carbs. For endomorphs in particular, who could be more susceptible to insulin resistance, this is quite helpful.

The Greatest Compound Workouts to Increase Muscle and Increase Metabolism

Incorporating complex workouts into your regimen is crucial to boosting muscle engagement and calorie expenditure. The following are a few of the top endomorphic compound movements:

A fundamental exercise that works the quads, hamstrings, glutes, and core is the squat. Goblet squats and front squats are two variations that can improve muscular engagement even more.

Deadlifts: This all-encompassing workout targets the back, legs, and core muscles. It works incredibly well to increase general strength and power.

Bench Press: A great upper-body exercise, the bench press targets the chest, shoulders, and triceps. Exercise variations that target different muscle fibers, such as incline and decline presses, can bring diversity.

Rows: Using barbells or dumbbells, rows work the back muscles efficiently, enhancing posture and encouraging a well-rounded body. They use the core to provide stability as well.

Endomorph Fat Loss Program

Overhead Press: This compound exercise strengthens the upper chest, triceps, and shoulders while requiring core stability. It also helps to develop upper-body strength.

These activities are perfect for endomorphs who want to reduce fat because they improve calorie burn while simultaneously helping you gain muscle.

9. Exercise Splits to Gain Muscle and Lose Fat

Endomorph Push-Pull-Legs (PPL) Workout (A/B Split Routine)

Endomorphs find that the Push-Pull-Legs (PPL) workout split works especially well since it maximizes recuperation while allowing for balanced training of all major muscle groups. Here's how to set up your PPL schedule:

On Push Day (A), concentrate on chest, shoulder, and triceps movements. Examples of tasks are as follows:

Bench Press
The Overhead Press
Dips
Dumbbell Press with an Incline
Pull Day (B): Use exercises like these to target your biceps and back.

Deadlifting
Pull-Ups
Overturned Rows

Endomorph Fat Loss Program

Pulls on faces

Leg Day (C): Focus on strengthening your lower body with drills such as these:

Squats

Lunges

Leg Press

Raising Calf

Cardio Integration: Low-Intensity Steady-State (LISS) and High-Intensity Interval Training (HIIT)

If you want to lose fat, you must include cardiovascular exercise in your routine. There are advantages to both HIIT and LISS:

High-intensity interval training, or HIIT, alternates brief bursts of vigorous exercise with rest intervals. HIIT works well and can help burn calories fast without sacrificing muscular mass. Typical HIIT activities could consist of:

Repeat for 20–30 minutes: 30 seconds of sprinting, followed by 1 minute of walking.

Low-Intensity Steady-State (LISS): This category comprises moderately paced swimming, cycling, and brisk walking. Longer sessions benefit from LISS, which can also be used to promote recovery following weight training or on days off.

Endomorphs can significantly improve cardiovascular health and expedite fat reduction by switching between HIIT and LISS.

Endomorph Fat Loss Program

Week-by-Week Progressive Workout Plan (Beginner, Intermediate, Advanced)

For further improvement, you must design an organized exercise program based on your current level of fitness. Here's an example weekly schedule:

Four-week Beginner Workout Plan:

Weeks 1-2: Concentrate on learning form while using smaller weights.
Push Day is on Monday (3 sets of 10–12 repetitions).
Pull Day is on Wednesday (3 sets of 10–12 repetitions).
It's Leg Day on Friday (3 sets of 10–12 reps).
Weeks 3–4: Increase weights gradually.
Monday: Push Day (3 sets of 8-10 reps)
Pull Day is on Wednesday (3 sets of 8–10 reps).
Leg Day is this Friday (3 sets of 8–10 reps).
Four-week Intermediate Workout Plan:

Weeks five and six: Include more exercises and variations.

Push Day is on Monday (4 sets of 8–10 reps).
Pull Day is on Wednesday (4 sets of 8–10 reps).
Leg Day is this Friday (4 sets of 8–10 reps).
Concentrate on progressive overload in weeks 7-8.

Push Day is on Monday (4 sets of 6–8 repetitions).

Endomorph Fat Loss Program

Pull Day is on Wednesday (4 sets of 6–8 reps).

Leg Day is on Friday (4 sets of 6–8 reps).

Four-week Advanced Workout Plan:

Weeks 9–10: Use sophisticated methods such as supersets.

It's Push Day on Monday (5 sets of 6–8 repetitions with supersets).

Tomorrow is Pull Day (5 sets of 6–8 repetitions plus supersets).

It's Leg Day on Friday (5 sets of 6–8 repetitions with supersets).

Week 11–12: Pay attention to maximum effort.

Monday is Push Day (four to six sets of reps).

Wednesday: Pull Day (5 sets of 4-6 reps)

Friday: Leg Day (four to six sets of repetitions)

Taking Care of Problem Areas: Hips, Thighs, and Belly

Try including these exercises to target areas that are prone to fat storage:

For the Belly: To strengthen the core and encourage abdominal definition, try planks, Russian twists, and hanging leg lifts.

For the Hips: Side lunges, hip thrusts, and glute bridges will help to tone the muscles while also strengthening the hips.

For the Thighs: To ensure balanced development, exercises like leg presses, step-ups, and squats will work the front and back of the thighs.

11. Getting Moving Outside of the Gym

Incorporating Functional Fitness and Everyday Movements

Exercise shouldn't be limited to the gym. Your overall health and fitness can be greatly improved by including regular exercises and functional fitness. The following are some tactics:

Exercises for functional fitness include lunges, pushups, and squats, which are movements that are representative of daily life. This increases flexibility and coordination in addition to strength.

Active Lifestyle: Make an effort to move more throughout the day. For short excursions, think about using the stairs rather than the elevator, walking or cycling, and pausing frequently during the day to stretch and stand up.

How to Stay Active During Days of Rest

Even while rest days are crucial for healing, you shouldn't be inactive. Here are some strategies for maintaining focus on days off:

Light Activity: Engage in light activities like walking, yoga, or swimming. This facilitates blood flow and speeds up healing without straining your muscles.

Endomorph Fat Loss Program

Active Hobbies: If you're looking for a hobby that requires you to move, try dancing, hiking, or sports. This is entertaining and soothing, and it can keep your moving.

Work on Flexibility and Mobility: Use foam rolling or stretching exercises to dedicate time to improving your range of motion and flexibility. This lessens discomfort and enhances the general quality of movement.

You may optimize your training regimen, encourage fat reduction, and develop a stronger, healthier physique that complements your endomorph objectives by using these components. Whether you're just starting or seeking to modify your approach, a well-structured fitness regimen combined with the correct diet can lead to revolutionary results.

Recall that achieving fitness involves more than just reaching your goal; it also entails accepting the trip and implementing long-lasting adjustments that improve your quality of life.

(SECTION 4:)

Endomorph Training Cheats and Techniques

12. The Mind-Muscle Connection: The Secret to Successful Exercise

How to Focus and Engage the Right Muscles During Exercise

Especially for endomorphs, one of the most critical components of resistance training is strengthening the mind-muscle link. In order to optimize muscle activation and make sure you're successfully targeting the targeted locations; this notion entails paying conscious attention to the muscle you're exercising during each exercise.

1. Techniques for Visualization: Take a moment to envision the muscle area you are working on before beginning any activity. When performing a bench press, for example, see the muscles in your chest contracting and relaxing with each repetition. This type of mental rehearsal increases muscular activation and improves focus.

Endomorph Fat Loss Program

2. Reduce the Speed of the Movement: By reducing the speed of your repetitions, you may experience all of the movement's phases, from the eccentric (falling) to the concentric (lifting). This enhances your technique and lengthens the period of time you are under tension, both of which can promote better fat loss and muscle gain.

3. Use Lighter Weights for Better Form: Although it may be tempting to lift larger weights, you can strengthen your connection with the muscles you are targeting by concentrating on lighter weights while keeping perfect form. For endomorphs in particular, this is very important because good form can guarantee effective muscle engagement and prevent injuries.

4. Use isometric holds while your movements are at their highest point. For example, during a bicep curl, pause for a second at the top of the curl to fully engage the biceps. Over time, this may improve muscle recruitment and lead to larger strength improvements.

You may improve your workouts and make sure you're really working the muscles required to reach your fitness objectives by concentrating on these approaches.

13. Lifting Techniques for Better Results

Posture corrections, appropriate form, and core bracing

Endomorph Fat Loss Program

For endomorphs in particular, who may be more prone to injuries and may find it difficult to maintain good form due to excess body fat, mastering lifting techniques is crucial. This is how to lift weights properly:

1. Core Bracing: For stability during any lift, your core must be engaged. Breathe deeply and contract your abdominal muscles as though you're about to land a punch to strengthen your core. This helps produce force during lifts and safeguards your spine. You can lift more weights and work out more quickly if you keep your core strong.

2. Correct Form: Form should always come before weight. Injuries can result from common errors like flaring your elbows during bench presses or rounding your back during deadlifts. Ensure that you:

For both squats and deadlifts, maintain a straight back and an erect chest.
To avoid putting stress on the joints, keep your knees in line with your toes.
Retain your wrists in a neutral position to prevent wrist pain.

3. Posture Corrections: Be mindful of your posture not only during physical activity but also at other times of the day. Your lifts may suffer from bad posture. Strengthening your upper back and shoulders through workouts like rows and face pulls will improve posture and boost your overall lifting technique.

Tricks to Make the Most of Every Workout

Endomorph Fat Loss Program

Exercises that target several muscle groups and increase calorie expenditure, such as squats, deadlifts, and bench presses, should be prioritized. Endomorphs, who need to maximize their training efficiency, can particularly benefit from this.

Watch Your Rest Times: It's important to give yourself enough time to recover between sets. For hypertrophy (muscle growth), aim for 30-90 seconds of rest, and for strength-focused sets, aim for 2-3 minutes. This equilibrium facilitates the preservation of intensity while permitting your muscles to recuperate for peak efficiency.

Employ Tempo Variations: Changing the tempo of your lifts can present fresh difficulties. Try, for instance, reducing the weight for three seconds during the eccentric phase and then lifting during the explosive concentric period. This method can encourage growth by stimulating muscle fibers in a new way.

Using these methods in your lifting regimen can improve performance and make working out more pleasurable. Remember, understanding the fundamentals is key for long-term success.

14. Cardiology for Endomorphs

What Kind and How Much Cardio Works Best?

Cardiovascular activity is essential for endomorphs looking to lose weight. However, depending on personal tastes and fitness levels, the kind and quantity of cardio can change.

Endomorph Fat Loss Program

1. The weekly target for duration and frequency of moderate-intensity aerobic activity should be 150–300 minutes. This can be divided into thirty-to-sixty-minute sessions. An alternative that works well is 75–150 minutes of high-intensity aerobic exercise.

2. Cardiovascular Types:

High-Intensity Interval Training (HIIT): Endomorphs benefit most from this. Short bursts of high intensity exercise are interspersed with rest or low intensity intervals in high-intensity training. As HIIT can enhance cardiovascular fitness and aid in weight loss, research indicates that it's a time-effective solution for people with hectic schedules.

Low-Intensity Steady-State (LISS): This category comprises steady-state swimming, cycling, and brisk walking. LISS is a great option for recuperation days and might be more pleasurable for those who would like work out with less impact.

For Maximum Fat Burn, Strike a Balance Between Strength and Endurance

For endomorphs, maintaining lean muscle mass while optimizing fat burn requires striking a balance between strength and cardio exercise. Here's how to attain this balance:

Combine Cardio with Resistance Training: Integrating cardio sessions into your strength training routine will maximize calorie burn and enhance recovery.

Endomorph Fat Loss Program

Think about adding brief cardio bursts (such as a 5-minute row) in between bouts of resistance training, or performing cardio after your strength training sessions.

Put Recovery First: Make sure you're giving yourself enough time to recover between strenuous aerobic and strength training sessions. Excessive training can cause weariness and impede development. Observe your body's cues and modify your regimen as necessary.

Pay Attention to Your Body: varied forms of strength and cardio training have varied effects on different people's bodies. Try out a variety of modalities and intensities to see what suits you the best.

Endomorphs can reach their fitness objectives more quickly by combining a strong strength training program with the appropriate kinds and quantities of cardio. The secret is to continue pushing yourself, be active, and have fun while you make the transition to a fitter, healthier lifestyle.

(SECTION 5:)

Maintaining Direction and Preventing Stagnation

15. Overcoming Typical Roadblocks

Managing Gradual Advancement and Weight-Loss Stalls

As an endomorph, starting a fat loss journey might be likened to a rollercoaster ride with ups and downs. Even while you might make great progress in the beginning, as you go along you might meet moderate progress or even a plateau. This is entirely normal and not just common. The key to your long-term success is knowing how to overcome these obstacles.

1. Acknowledging Plateaus: Recognizing that they are an inevitable aspect of the process is the first step in getting past a weight-loss plateau. Your body may become more adept at using energy as it adjusts to your new lifestyle, which could cause your weight to drop more slowly. Remember that life isn't always a straight line and that it's acceptable to go through phases of change.

2. Analyzing Your Routine: Examine your diet and workout routine carefully if you find yourself at a standstill. Have you strayed from your original plan, or

Endomorph Fat Loss Program

are you still sticking to it? Reigniting fat loss can occasionally be achieved by making little adjustments to your macronutrient ratios, cutting back on calories somewhat, or intensifying your workouts.

For instance, to test your muscles in different ways, if you've been performing steady-state cardio, think about adding HIIT or altering your strength training regimen.

3. Concentrate on Non-Scale Victories: When the scale remains unchanged, it can be easy to lose hope, but attempt to direct your attention toward other signs of advancement. Do your clothes fit you better now? Have you seen gains in your endurance or strength? Do you have more energy now? Honoring these non-scale successes can keep you motivated and provide you a more comprehensive picture of your development.

Tips for Staying Motivated on a Mental and Emotional Level

Weight loss involves both physical and psychological components, and both are crucial. The following tactics will assist you in staying motivated and continuing forward motion:

1. Establish Small, Achievable Goals: Divide your journey into smaller, more attainable objectives rather than concentrating just on the overall picture. This might be as easy as deciding to lift a greater weight, start a new exercise regimen, or strive to lose a specific number of pounds each month. Rejoicing in these tiny successes can boost your motivation and give you a sense of success.

Endomorph Fat Loss Program

2. Establish a Support System: Whether it's family, friends, or a workout partner, surround yourself with people who encourage you to reach your goals. Share your hardships and triumphs with them. Sometimes all you need to get through difficult times is the knowledge that someone else is supporting you.

3. Journaling: Maintaining a journal can be a very effective way to reflect on and stay motivated. Keep track of your meals, exercise routine, and emotional condition as you go. This enables you to recognize trends and recognize your accomplishments, no matter how modest.

4. Engage in self-compassion and mindfulness exercises: treating yourself with kindness is crucial throughout this process. Gaining and losing weight is a journey, and setbacks are common. Including mindfulness exercises like yoga or meditation might help you become more resilient mentally and cope with stress better.

16. Monitoring Your Development

Using Strength Gains, Measurements, and Pictures as Markers

Monitoring your progress is essential for keeping you motivated and confirming that you're headed in the right direction. In addition to using the scale, you can track your progress using these numerous efficient methods:

1. Body Measurements: Taking measurements of your arms, thighs, hips, and waist can provide you important information about how much muscle you've gained and lost. To monitor improvements over time, think about taking

measurements every four weeks. Even in cases where there aren't any appreciable changes on the scale, many people discover that their body composition improves.

2. development Pictures: Having regular pictures of your development might act as a visual reminder of your advancements. Try to get shots with comparable lighting and perspectives so you can track small changes in your body over time. These visual cues can be quite inspiring, particularly if the scale doesn't display results right away.

3. Strength increases: Tracking your strength increases with a training journal can provide you a concrete indicator of your development. Are you lifting larger weights or accomplishing more reps? One of the most important signs that your training program is working is when you see gains in your strength and endurance.

4. Fitness examinations: Consider doing frequent fitness examinations that measure endurance, flexibility, and general performance. Timed runs, push-up challenges, and flexibility evaluations are a few examples of exercises that can help you determine your general level of fitness and highlight areas for growth.

How to Modify Your Initiative for Ongoing Outcomes

The next step is to modify your program as necessary to guarantee ongoing outcomes after you've set up a system to monitor your progress. Here are some tactics to think about:

Endomorph Fat Loss Program

1. Vary Your Exercises: Your body may have adapted if you have been doing the same exercise regimen for a long time. Occasionally switch up your workouts to prevent plateaus. This might be experimenting with different workout forms (such as circuit training, supersets, or modifying your cardio), adding new exercises, or changing your rep ranges.

2. Modify Your Diet: Your calorie requirements will fluctuate as you shed pounds. Make sure your calorie intake and macronutrient breakdown are in line with your current objectives by regularly assessing them. To continue improving, you might need to cut back on calories a little or adjust your macronutrient ratios.

3. Listen to Your Body: Pay attention to how your body responds to your regimen. It might be time to reevaluate your training volume, intensity, or recovery techniques if you're feeling worn out or uncomfortable. For long-term success, recuperation days must be prioritized and enough sleep must be obtained.

4. Consider Professional help: If you find yourself failing to make progress despite your best efforts, getting help from a trained fitness professional or a registered dietitian can provide personalized insights. By creating a program specifically for you, they can assist you in overcoming challenges and achieving your objectives.

(Section 6:)

A Long-Term Strategy for Fat Loss

17. Preserving Your Outcomes

Making the Switch from Losing Weight to Maintaining Muscle

Best wishes. As an endomorph, you have accomplished a huge feat if you have reached a position where you have lost a large amount of weight. But losing weight is just the first step in the process; maintaining your muscle mass and long-term fat loss are equally important to maintaining your gains. To avoid gaining back fat and maintain your hard-earned muscle, you must approach this phase strategically by striking a balance between your dietary requirements and workout routine.

1. Setting New Objectives: It's critical to reevaluate your objectives after you've reached your desired weight. Rather than concentrating only on weight loss, make it a priority to maintain your present body type while increasing or retaining muscle mass. You may maintain your motivation and interest in your fitness journey by adopting this mental shift.

2. Changing Your Calorie Intake: Your body needs less calories to maintain your current weight after weight loss than it did when you were heavier. Find a maintenance level that is suitable for you and gradually increase your calorie intake. Throughout this shift, keep a careful eye on your weight; in many cases,

Endomorph Fat Loss Program

a modest daily calorie increase of 100–200 will be enough to sustain your new weight without gaining weight.

3. Stressing Protein: As you shift to maintaining your muscle mass, continue to consume a lot of protein. Protein is essential for building and repairing muscles, especially if you keep up your resistance exercise regimen. Depending on your level of exercise, aim for 1.2 to 2.2 grams of protein per kilogram of body weight.

4. Sustaining a Balanced Macronutrient Profile: Despite the allure of consuming more carbohydrates after losing weight, it's important to keep your diet balanced. Focus on a diet rich in lean proteins, healthy fats, and complex carbohydrates. This well-rounded strategy not only helps to maintain muscular mass but also improves general health.

5. Remaining Active: Maintain your regular exercise schedule, emphasizing a mix of aerobic and resistance training exercises. Cardiovascular exercises will help you burn any surplus calories and maintain muscle mass. Resistance training will help you maintain muscle mass.

How to Add Carbs Back in Without Putting on Weight

It can be difficult to reintroduce carbohydrates following a weight loss phase, particularly for endomorphs who may be more likely to gain weight. You may, however, enjoy carbohydrates and yet achieve your goals if you plan ahead and eat mindfully.

Endomorph Fat Loss Program

1. Reintroduction Gradually: Reintroduce carbohydrates into your meals gradually rather than returning abruptly to a high-carb diet. To begin, incorporate tiny servings of complex carbohydrates into your meals, like quinoa, brown rice, or sweet potatoes, and observe the effects on your body. By using this strategy, you can prevent unexpected weight gain.

2. Timing Is Everything: Be mindful of when you eat carbohydrates. It can be very helpful to time your carbohydrate intake in relation to your exercise. Consuming carbohydrates both before and after exercise gives your body energy throughout training and facilitates recuperation afterward.

3. Put Whole Foods First: When reintroducing carbohydrates, give preference to whole, nutrient-dense foods over processed ones. The high fiber, vitamin, and mineral content of whole meals can help with blood sugar regulation and digestion.

4. Track Your Progress: Keep a record of your weight and body measurements as you reintroduce carbohydrates. You should modify your carbohydrate consumption if you start to gain weight unintentionally. You can discover the ideal balance for your body with the aid of this monitoring.

5. Watch Your Portion Sizes: Consuming too many carbohydrates might rapidly result in consuming too many calories. By observing portion sizes, paying attention to your body's hunger cues, and abstaining from mindless snacking, you can practice mindful eating.

18. Endomorphs and Health Throughout Life

Choosing a Sustainable Way of Living Outside of the Program

A sustainable lifestyle is essential to obtaining long-term health as you strive to preserve your results. This stage is more about striking a balance that works for your life than it is about rigorous dieting or excessive activity.

1. Put Balance Above Perfection: Acknowledge that living a healthy lifestyle doesn't have to be flawless. Give yourself permission to indulge occasionally without feeling bad about it. Moderation is the key. Long-term adherence can be facilitated by a comprehensive approach to nutrition and exercise.

2. Make Healthy Habits a Routine: Consistency is key for retaining outcomes. Include healthful practices in your everyday routine, such as planning meals in advance, exercising frequently, and placing a high priority on rest and sleep. Establishing routines helps to make healthy living more fun and easier to maintain.

3. Take Part in Physical Activities You Love: Whether it's dancing, hiking, cycling, or group fitness courses, choose physical activities you truly enjoy. Maintaining an active and healthy lifestyle is simpler when you enjoy what you do.

4. Remain informed: wisdom is strength. Continue your education regarding fitness, diet, and overall well-being. This knowledge will empower you to make informed choices and change your lifestyle as needed.

Endomorph Fat Loss Program

5. Seek Assistance: Establishing a network of support is critical to long-term success. Be in the company of loved ones, friends, or online groups that have similar objectives. Giving others access to your experiences, setbacks, and victories may inspire and hold people accountable.

Managing a Healthy Metabolism Over Time

For endomorphs, keeping a healthy metabolism is essential, particularly when considering long-term health. The following tactics can help you maintain an ideal metabolism:

1. Make Strength Training a Priority: One of the best strategies to increase your metabolism is to perform strength training on a regular basis. Maintaining and increasing muscle mass is essential for protecting metabolic health because muscle burns more calories at rest than fat.

2. Keep Moving Throughout the Day: Find methods to add extra activity to your everyday schedule in addition to your scheduled workouts. Simple actions like walking during breaks, using the stairs instead of the elevator, or taking up active hobbies can all contribute to this.

3. Control Stress: Prolonged stress can impair your metabolism. Utilize stress-reduction methods like yoga, meditation, or deep breathing exercises to maintain metabolic health and control cortisol levels.

Endomorph Fat Loss Program

4. Make Sure You Get Enough Sleep: Because good sleep is so important to metabolic health, make it a priority. Aim for 7-9 hours of restful sleep per night. Hormonal imbalances brought on by sleep deprivation may have an impact on metabolism and appetite.

5. Keep Yourself Hydrated: Adequate hydration can aid in metabolic processes and is crucial for general health. Try to be well-hydrated throughout the day because a dehydrated body can have a slower metabolism and less energy.

6. Reassess Your Goals Frequently: As you move into a long-term maintenance phase, review your objectives frequently and modify your strategy as necessary. Your approach to fitness and health may need to alter as life does.

Endomorph Fat Loss Program

Developing lasting practices that support lifetime health and well-being is a more sustainable method to fat loss for endomorphs than simply losing weight. You can succeed in your health journey by sustaining your results with a supportive lifestyle, consistent exercise, and mindful eating. Accept the adjustments you've made, acknowledge your accomplishments, and remain dedicated to a well-rounded strategy that enables you to have the healthiest possible life. Even if the path may present obstacles, you can attain long-lasting outcomes and lead an active, satisfying life if you are persistent and use the appropriate techniques.

Conclusion: Highlighting Your Achievements and Celebrating Your Success
Now that this chapter of your adventure to discovering and maximizing your endomorphic body type has come to an end, take a moment to acknowledge and appreciate the amazing progress you have accomplished. Every improvement, regardless of whether it's weight loss, muscular growth, or just adopting healthier habits, should be acknowledged. This journey is about more than just changing your physical appearance; it's about accepting a new way of thinking, finding your inner power, and laying the foundation for long-term wellness.

Consider Your Journey Again

Endomorph Fat Loss Program

The road to fitness and health is frequently paved with setbacks and victories. Being an endomorph, you might have encountered certain difficulties that called for tenacity and resolve. Maybe you experienced difficulties with weight swings or became irritated with the scale's intransigence. You now know how to sort through a sea of contradicting advice regarding exercises and diets to come up with a plan that works for you. Your devotion to knowing your body and its unique needs is shown in every choice you make, from diet planning to exercise regimens.

Celebrate all of your accomplishments, no matter how tiny. In the gym, did you set a new personal best? Have you felt happier and more energized lately? Perhaps you've come to like preparing nutritious meals rather than grabbing fast food. These successes signify a change in your way of thinking and living, not just a passing fancy.

Creating New Routines

The new behaviors you've developed are the foundation of your success. You now understand the significance of finding the ideal macronutrient balance for your particular body composition. Your dedication to strength training and exercise has given you the ability to take charge of your metabolism, demonstrating the extraordinary adaptability of the human body. Recall that creating and maintaining new behaviors is the cornerstone of long-lasting change.

1. You've adopted a consistent approach to your exercise and diet, realizing that long-term outcomes are the consequence of consistent effort. This devotion is

Endomorph Fat Loss Program

what differentiates those who thrive from those who struggle. Every time you put your health first, you feed a constructive feedback loop that moves you ahead.

2. Accepting a Growth mentality: You have learned to accept a growth mentality as a result of this adventure. You understand that obstacles are a necessary component of growth and do not define who you are. Every obstacle you encounter presents an opportunity for growth and adaptation, fostering resilience that will benefit you in all facets of your life.

Creating Future Objectives

It's time to focus on the future now that you have a solid foundation in place. Think about the next thing you wish to achieve. Perhaps you want to try out some new healthy dishes, learn a new activity, or increase your cardiovascular fitness. These ambitions will keep you motivated and interested as you continue your path.

1. Customize Your Goals: Make sure your goals reflect your hobbies and way of life. Whether you want to compete in a local fitness competition or simply enjoy outdoor sports with friends, setting your goals can offer you direction and purpose.

2. Recall that progress is not always linear and instead should be the primary focus. You can experience setbacks or plateaus as you proceed. Accept these times as a chance to rethink your strategy and make the required corrections.

Endomorph Fat Loss Program

Appreciate the little victories you have along the road since they add to your total achievement.

Think about the value of a supporting community as you proceed on your health path. Being around by others who share your values may inspire, uplift, and hold you accountable. Making connections with people who share your aims, whether through local health clubs, online forums, or fitness courses, can improve your experience and forge enduring friendships.

1. Talk About Your Journey: Don't be afraid to let people know about your achievements and setbacks. Someone else going through similar struggles might find inspiration in your tale, and the support you get might be priceless.

2. Seek Advice: Take into account consulting a coach or enrolling in an endomorph-specific exercise regimen. Professional assistance can give insights and tactics that increase your progress, providing a fresh perspective on your journey.

Success over the long haul demands constant dedication and flexibility. Be receptive to fresh perspectives on your fitness and well-being as you proceed. Engage both your body and intellect in the process by persistently searching out events and information that will improve your life.

B. TERZA 54

Endomorph Fat Loss Program

1. Review Your Plan Frequently: As your wants and objectives change, so do your needs in life. Make sure your diet and exercise regimens are still in line with your changing goals by regularly reviewing them. This adaptability will enable you to focus on your health and adjust to changes in life.

2. Make self-care a priority. Being healthy and fit involves more than just going to the gym and cooking. Make self-care routines that support mental and emotional health a priority. Fostering your general well-being is crucial, whether it is through hobbies, meditation, or spending time with close friends and family.

Last Words

As you take stock of your achievements, keep in mind that this is a lifelong commitment to health and happiness rather than a final destination. Honor the successes, draw lessons from the setbacks, and look forward to the path ahead. You have the abilities, know-how, and fortitude to design a lively, happy, and energetic life.

You've set yourself up for long-term success by accepting your particular body type, being aware of your nutritional requirements, and making the commitment to live a sustainable lifestyle. You are at the beginning of an unending journey filled with possibilities. Proceed, rejoice in your accomplishments, and never stop motivating people around you. You have incredible potential, and the best is still to come!

CALL TO ACTION

Thank you for reading!

I'd like to personally thank you for taking the time to read my work. I really appreciate your time and effort, and I hope this book has provided you with valuable success tools and insights.

Your feedback is really useful to me as I grow as a writer. I would love to hear your feedback, whether positive or negative, so that I may develop and make future works even more useful and fascinating.

I humbly request that you offer an honest review if you found this book worthwhile or if you believe anything may be improved. Your counsel will help me not only improve, but also become a better person.

Thank you again for your support, and I look forward to hearing from you!

SINCERLY